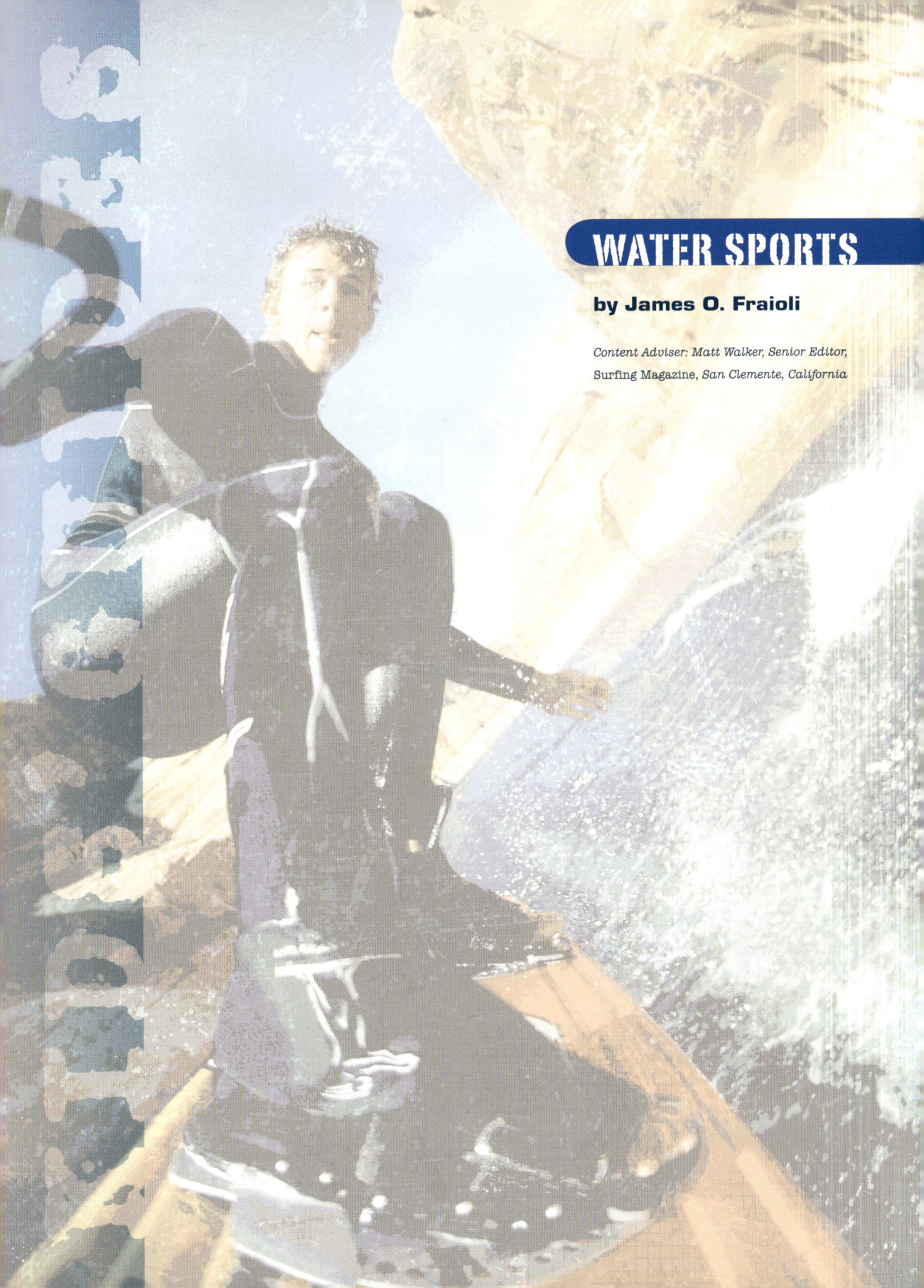

WATER SPORTS

by James O. Fraioli

*Content Adviser: Matt Walker, Senior Editor,
Surfing Magazine, San Clemente, California*

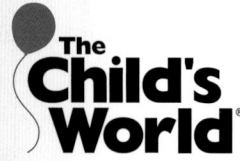

Published in the United States of America by The Child's World®
PO Box 326 • Chanhassen, MN 55317-0326 • 800-599-READ • www.childsworld.com

Acknowledgments

The Child's World®: Mary Berendes, Publishing Director

Editorial Directions, Inc.: E. Russell Primm, Editorial Director; Melissa McDaniel, Line Editor; Matt Messbarger, Project Editor and Editorial Assistant; Susan Hindman, Copy Editor; Susan Ashley, Proofreader; Terry Johnson, Olivia Nellums, Katharine Trickle, and Julie Zaveloff, Fact Checkers; Tim Griffin/IndexServ, Indexer; James Buckley Jr. and James Gigliotti, Photo Researchers and Selectors

Editorial and photo research services provided by Shoreline Publishing Group LLC, Santa Barbara, California

The Design Lab: Kathleen Petelinsek, Art Direction and Design; Kari Thornborough, Art Production

Photos

Cover: Corbis; AP/Wide World: 28; Jim Arbogast/Corbis: 12; Bettmann/Corbis: 7; Jonathan Blair/Corbis: 19; Paula Bronstein/Getty Images: 11; Corbis: 8; Rick Doyle/Corbis: 22; Mark Johnson/Corbis: 9; George Lepp/Corbis: 17; Chris Polk/WireImage: 26; Neil Rabinowitz/Corbis: 14; ReutersNewMedia/Corbis: 24; Grafton Smith/Corbis: 5; Sports Gallery/Al Messerschmidt: 21.

Registration

Copyright © 2005 by The Child's World®. All rights reserved.
No part of this book may be reproduced or utilized in any form or by any means without written permission from the publisher.

Library of Congress Cataloging-in-Publication Data

Fraioli, James O., 1968-
 Water sports / by James O. Fraioli.
   v. cm. — (Kids' guides)
 Includes bibliographical references and index.
 Contents: Water sport pioneers—Gearing up for action—Hit the water!—Stars and competition.
 ISBN 1-59296-212-2 (Library bound : alk. paper) 1. Aquatic sports—Juvenile literature.
[1. Aquatic sports.] I. Title. II. Series.
 GV770.5.F73 2004
 797—dc22   2003027367

KIDS' GUIDES TO EXTREME SPORTS: Water Sports

CONTENTS

4 introduction
Wild Fun on the Water

6 chapter one
Water Sports Pioneers

11 chapter two
Gearing Up for Action

16 chapter three
Hit the Water!

24 chapter four
Stars and Competition

30 glossary

31 find out more

32 index

INTRODUCTION

WILD FUN ON THE WATER

Have you ever seen people surfing at the beach or skipping on skis behind a boat? Have you ever said, "That could be me"? If so, now's the time to try a water sport!

More than 30 million people water-ski and wakeboard, while millions of others surf, bodyboard, kneeboard, windsurf, kitesurf, and **hydrofoil** surf. With so many sports to choose from, the hardest part might be deciding which one is right for you.

Water sports used to be limited to swimming or boating. But today's water-lovers have taken the fun and wild action of the street—such as skateboarding and stunt bike riding—to the world of water. This book looks at the coolest, most extreme water sports around.

If you like to swim, then you will like water sports. But make no mistake—they can be dangerous if you aren't familiar with the sport. All beginners should take lessons. Lessons help you learn how to do it—and how to do it safely. As you get better, you might want to enter competitions. Thousands of them take place across the country all summer long.

So choose a water sport that interests you. After

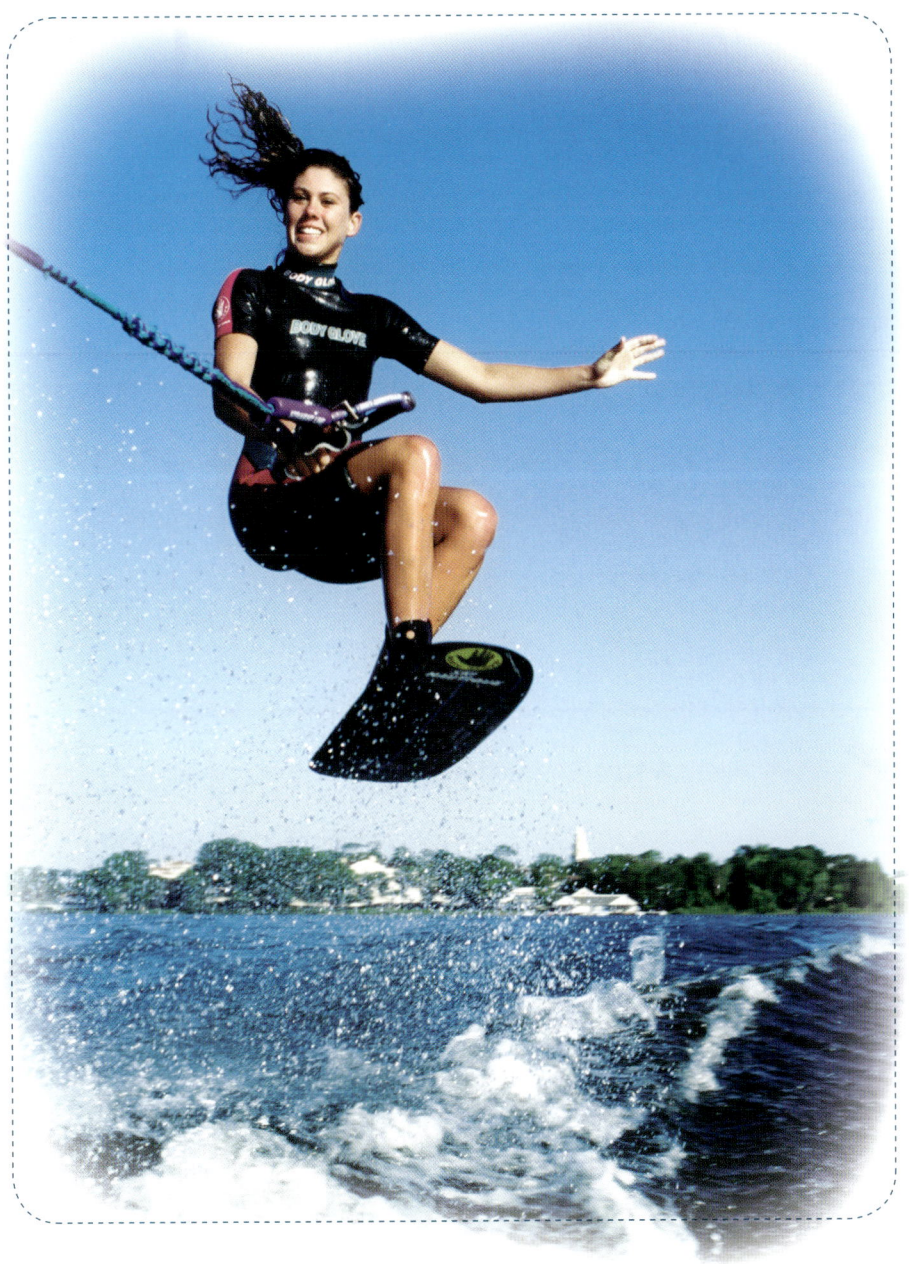

High-flying wakeboard action is just one of many ways you can have fun on the water.

some lessons and practice, you'll be catching a perfect wave,

waterskiing barefoot, or racing across a lake powered by

the wind!

CHAPTER one

WATER SPORTS PIONEERS

Using technology, daring, and the power of nature, water sports lovers have come up with many action-packed ways to play in the waves.

Surf and Ski

Today's surfers are carrying on a long tradition. Ancient rock carvings tell the stories of great surfing feats as far back as 1500, and the sport may have begun even earlier.

Water-skiers got started a bit more recently. The first person to water-ski was 18-year-old Ralph Samuelson from Minnesota, who, in 1922, strapped on a pair of snow skis and hit the water. Later, he boiled two 8-foot (2.4-meter) wooden planks to soften them, curved the tips, and used leather for bindings. Three years later, Fred Waller designed his own pair of water skis. Samuelson took Waller's invention a leap ahead by riding his planks over a homemade jump ramp.

In 1939, Jack Andersen invented the trick ski so he could perform stunts, adding more excitement to the sport of waterskiing. Eight years later, Dick Pope Jr. invented barefoot skiing—zipping over the water using just your feet—eliminating skis altogether.

In the early 1960s, freeboarding was developed as a

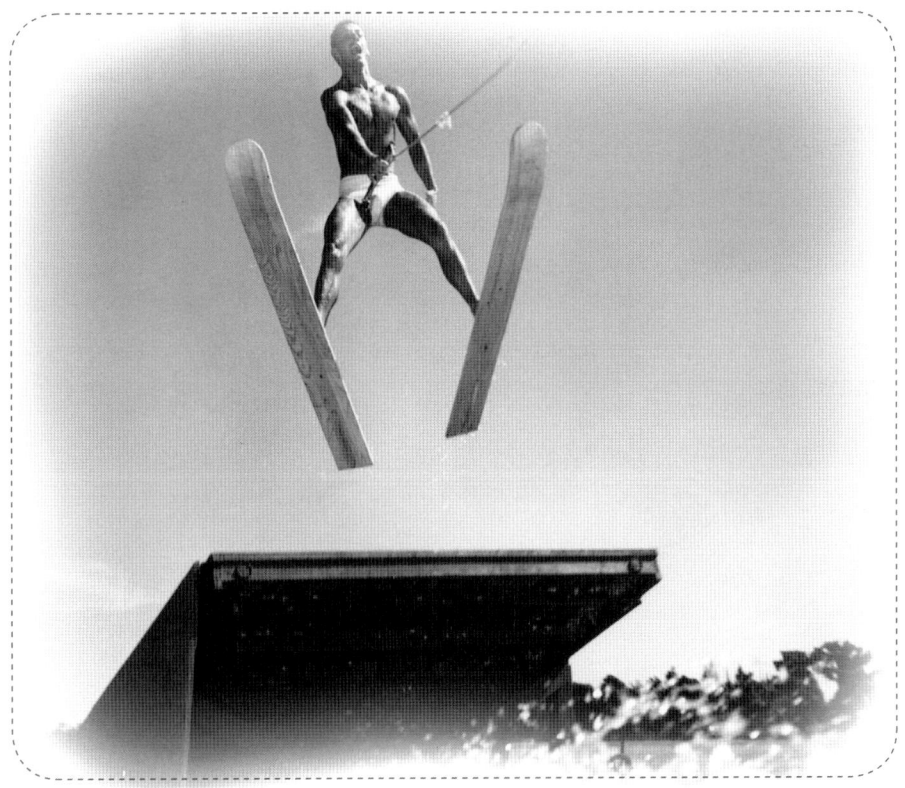

Early water-skiers always used two skis, which were much wider than today's models.

way for surfers to get out on their boards on days when the water was too flat to do any surfing. Freeboarding refers to the act of riding a surfboard that's connected to a boat, similar to waterskiing.

During the late 1960s and early 1970s, three California surfers built themselves homemade kneeboards and bodyboards to be towed behind a boat. From these, shorter boards developed, and water sports got even cooler. Then, in 1985, San Diego surfer Tony Finn came up with the skurfer, or wakeboard, which he used to combine surfing and waterskiing. In wakeboarding, riders use the boat's **wake** to launch themselves into the air to do tricks.

Harnessing the Wind

In 1948, 20-year-old Newman Darby wanted something totally different in a water sport. He designed a handheld sail mounted on a small **catamaran.** Californians Jim Drake (a sailor)

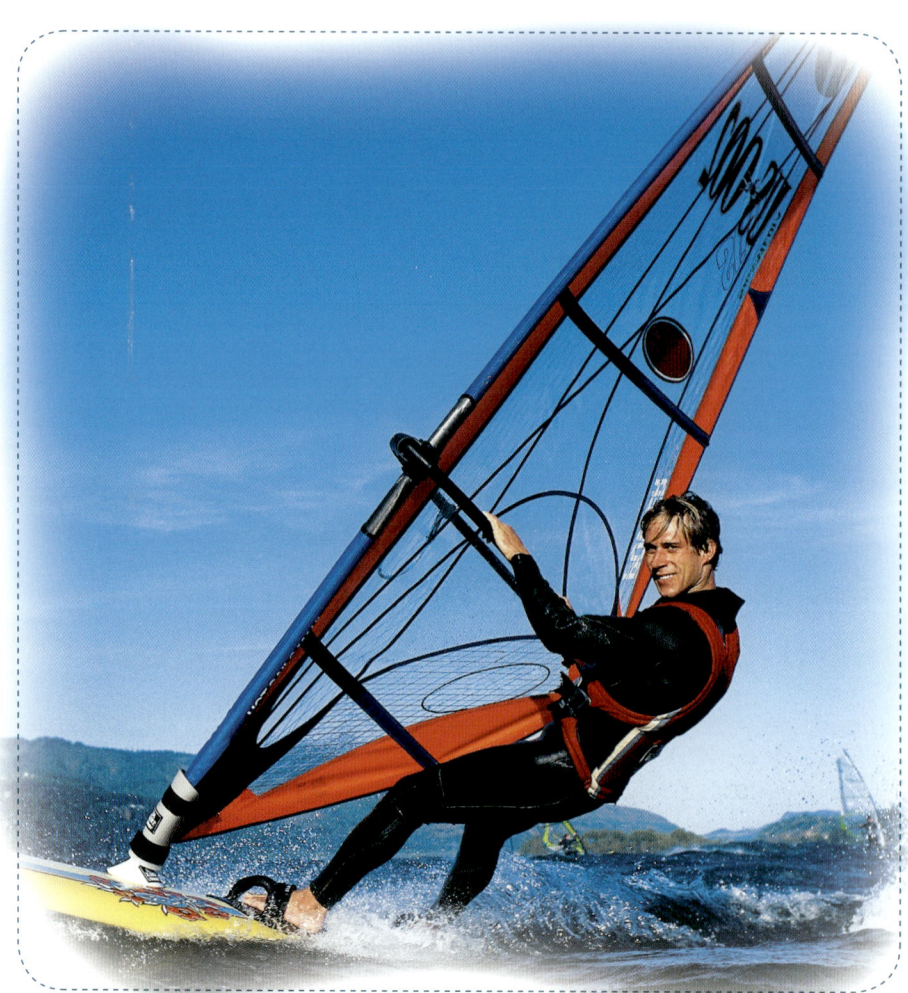

Windsurfing combines the wind power of sailing with the wave-riding action of surfing.

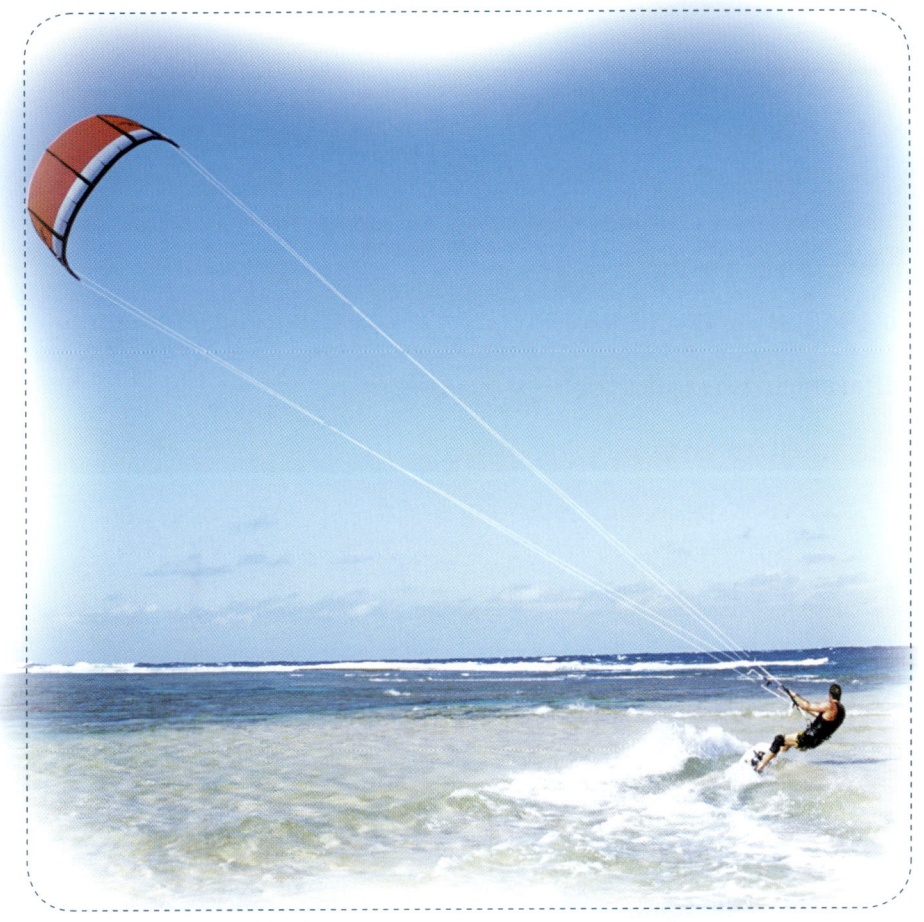

Kitesurfing is one of the newest water sports—and perhaps the fastest moving!

and Hoyle Schweitzer (a surfer) designed a similar sailboard in 1968. They called their creation a windsurfer. To windsurf, you stand on a board and zoom across (or over!) the waves using the power of wind in the sail.

Looking for an even greater thrill, Cory Roeseler from Oregon came up with a KiteSki system in the 1980s. At the same time in France, the Legaignoux brothers were working on their flysurf system. Both of these ideas led to kitesurfing,

NO SURFING IN HAWAII?

Beginning in 1890, surfing in Hawaii nearly became extinct. Christian missionaries wanted to change Hawaiian culture by getting rid of traditions such as hula dancing and surfing. They even tried outlawing surfing, among other things. The sport was slowly dying out in the very islands where it was born.

It wasn't until the 1920s that Hawaiian athlete Duke Kahanamoku helped revive interest in surfing in Hawaii and elsewhere. Kahanamoku was one of the world's best swimmers. He had won the 100-meter freestyle gold medals in the 1912 and 1920 Olympics. His popularity helped him bring surfing to the rest of the United States. He gave demonstrations of the sport on long, wooden boards. Surfing quickly caught on, especially in Southern California.

which Laird Hamilton and Manu Bertin popularized in Hawaii in the 1990s. In this sport, a huge, nylon kite flying high above the waves pulls riders through the water.

Bob Woolley and his then-partner Mike Murphy invented the first sit-down hydrofoil water ski—a suspended chair with ski attachments that zips over the water. It went on sale to the public in 1989. With the hydrofoil, the board no longer meets the water. The early foilboard (as it's also called) had blunt, bulky edges and huge fins. Its top speed was only 17 miles (27 kilometers) per hour. As riders skills improved, so did the foilboard, and today, a whole new group of hydrofoil surfers takes to the waves.

CHAPTER **two**

GEARING UP FOR ACTION

To participate in water sports you need

good upper body strength, loads of **stamina,** and lessons from a qualified instructor. Every water sport can be dangerous, it's important to know your own limits so you won't get hurt. Using the right equipment is also important to enjoying water sports safely. Most people start with lessons where the equipment is provided. You can also rent before you buy.

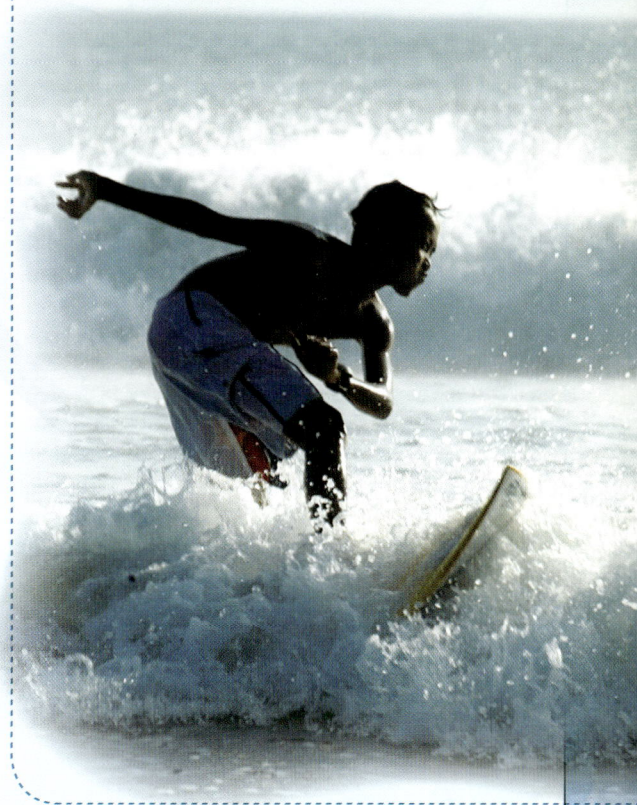

Little kids can catch great waves, too, even if just in the whitewater near shore.

Surfing/Bodyboarding

For the beginning surfer, a foamie is the right board to choose. A foamie is long, wide, and **buoyant,** giving you the best chance of remaining balanced once you are on your feet.

After you have practiced with a foamie, you will be ready to rent or buy your first board. You have a lot of choices when buying a board. They come in many different lengths and weights. Talk to local surfers about what is the best board for you, and make sure to try out many styles of

11

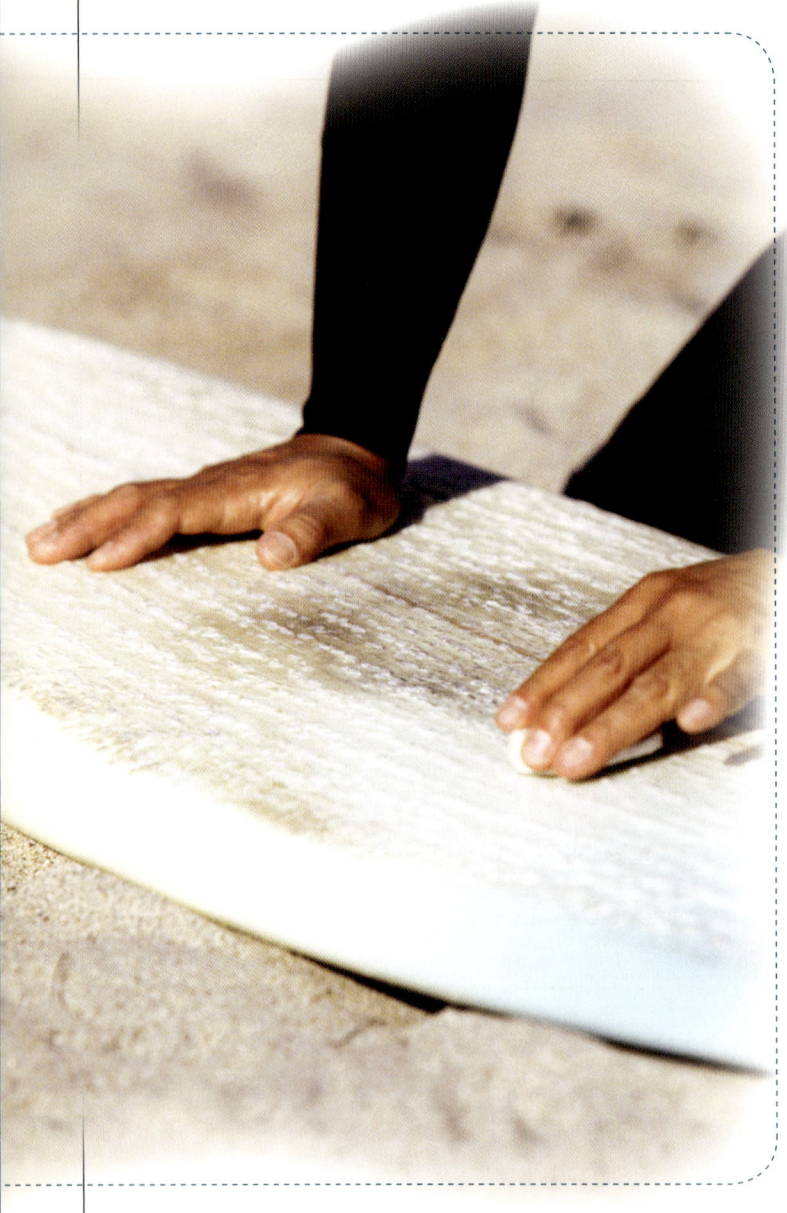

Getting ready to surf means waxing the board to create a good grip for your feet.

boards before you buy one. Find out about the types of waves in your area.

You'll also need surf wax, which is spread on top of the board to provide a grip for your feet. Always wax the board before getting into the water. Use soft wax for cold water and harder wax for warm water. You might also want to get a traction pad. It's a piece of foam traction for your back foot that sticks on the deck of the surfboard.

Another item you'll want is a leash. One end of the leash is attached to the board, the other around your ankle. The leash keeps you and the board together when you wipe out (fall off the board).

Depending on the temperature of the water, you may need a wet suit. A wet suit is made from neoprene rubber and works by trapping a layer of water between the suit and your body. The water then is warmed up by your body heat and keeps you from getting cold.

Like surfing, bodyboarding is very popular. For most new riders, catching a wave with a bodyboard (sometimes called a boogie board) is easier than surfing. You ride a bodyboard, which is shorter and lighter than a surfboard, lying on your stomach. Along with the bodyboard, you will need a pair of bodyboard fins. Fins will help you get past the breaking waves and give you that kick-start you need to catch a wave and ride it as it is breaking.

Waterskiing/Kneeboarding/Wakeboarding

For these sports, you need access to a speedboat, since they all involve being pulled over a calm ocean or lake. You might also need a wet suit, depending on the temperature of the water.

Besides the boat, a nonstretch ski rope with a handle is a must. It is also important that you wear a **life vest** at all times.

You can rent or buy water skis. After mastering two skis, you'll be ready to try one ski, then the shorter, wider trick skis, then jump skis, and eventually no skis!

Kneeboarding, in which you kneel while being pulled behind the boat, is similar to waterskiing. It requires a single board with a foam pad.

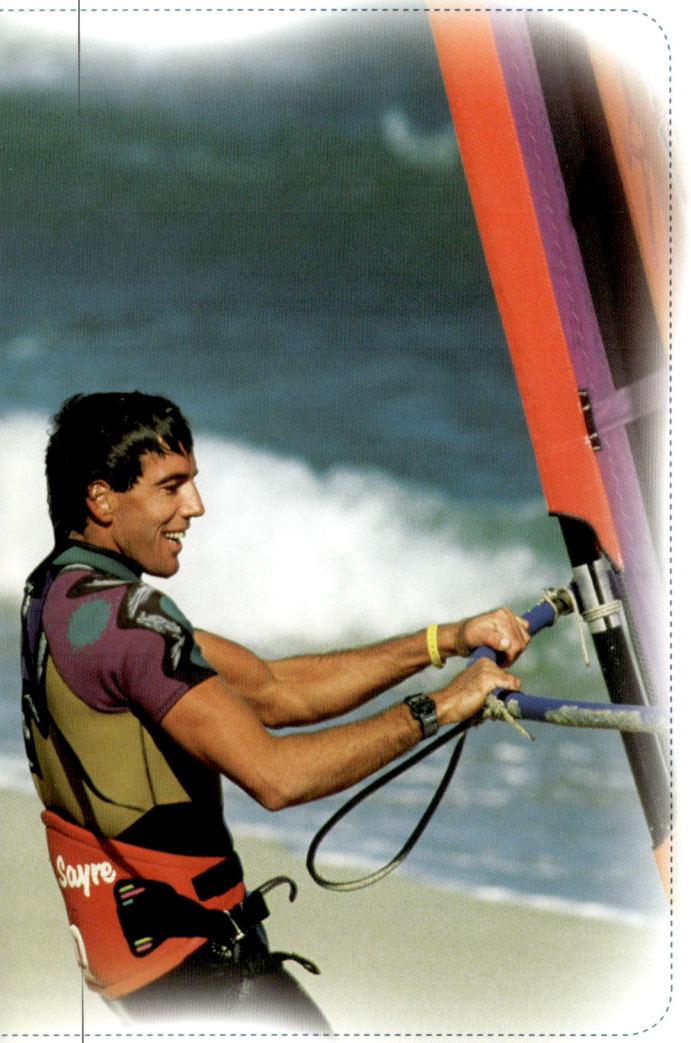

Windsurfing gear includes a harness (red gear), the boom (what he is holding), and the sail.

Wakeboarding uses a board that you strap your feet into. As the boat pulls you, you stand on the board and "surf" over the boat's wake.

Windsurfing/ Kitesurfing/Hydrofoil Surfing

Most good windsurfing schools will provide you with a board, usually one about 11 feet (3.4 m) long. Pick a board buoyant enough to allow you to stand and balance. The lighter you are, the shorter the board you can use.

Kitesurfing is a combination of kite flying, windsurfing, and wakeboarding. First, you'll need a kite—not the kind you fly in a park, but one made especially for this sport. You'll also need a wet suit, board,

> **FIRST-AID STOP**
>
> Water sports are so much fun it's hard to think of them as athletic activities, but they are—and they take place in dangerous environments. Here are some tips on avoiding injuries:
> - Exercise regularly.
> - Always wear a life vest or flotation device.
> - Never perform the sport alone. Always have a buddy with you. Try to enter the water at places where lifeguards are watching.
> - Make sure you get plenty of rest before hitting the water.
> - Make eating a healthy diet part of your lifestyle.
> - Wear sunblock. Even if you have a deep, dark tan, sunblock will help prevent **skin cancer.**
> - If you get hurt, tell your parents or an adult and see a doctor.

harness, and helmet. Kitesurfing is an expensive sport. You can save money by converting an old surfboard into a kiteboard by adding foot straps. This will work well as a learning board, but after you become more skilled, you'll want to buy a commercial kiteboard.

For hydrofoil surfers, or foilboarders, there are two types of boards on the market: the Sky Ski and the Air Chair. Hydrofoils are very expensive, but they can also be used while kitesurfing, behind a boat, or attached to a windsurfer. Hydrofoils can also be used in an ocean or a lake. Other hydrofoil equipment includes a helmet, leash, ski rope, and handle.

CHAPTER three

HIT THE WATER!

After you've taken lessons, it's time

to practice what you have learned. Before getting wet, learn about the water you'll be in. Talk to someone who is familiar with the wind direction, **water current,** and the dangers of where you are going. For instance, if you are windsurfing, you will **drift,** like any boat, downwind or with the current. That is why you should ask yourself, "What is down there?" If "down there" is a swamp with water snakes, you might not want to sail in that spot.

Before you start, always make sure you have a partner. Aside from helping you if you get hurt, a partner will keep you happy when you get frustrated and will make the sport more fun.

Surfing/Bodyboarding

To find a place to surf, go to your nearest surf shop and ask people where a good wave break is for beginners. This is not the time to pretend you're better than you are—some surf spots should only be attempted by real experts.

Before paddling out, sit and watch the surf. Watch what people are doing. Where is everybody sitting? Where do they paddle out?

Next, wax your board. Put the leash on what will be your back leg when you are riding a wave. Walk your board out until the water is waist deep and then hop on. Start by lying face-down on the board. Then try sitting up, with your legs in the water. Position your body on the board so that the board's nose is barely out of the water. After paddling out, watch what others are doing. Then get ready.

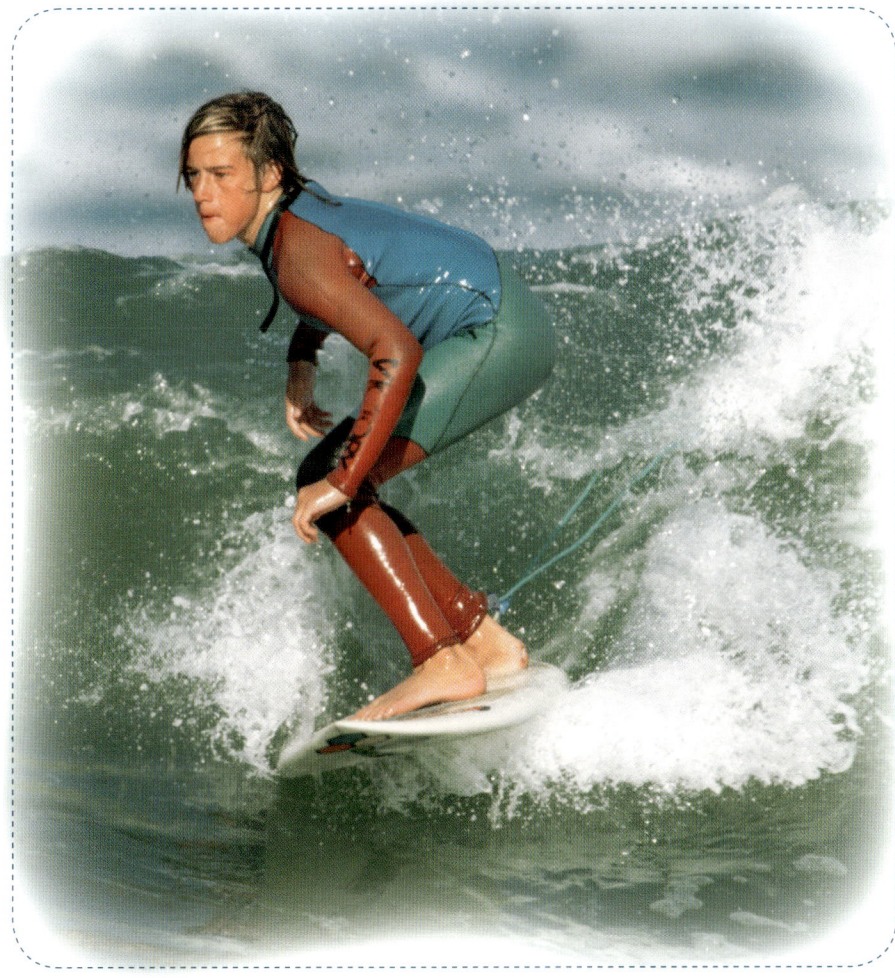

After picking out a wave, a surfer stands up and rides the waves toward shore.

Knowing which wave to paddle for, which to let pass, and when to start paddling are things no one can teach you. They will come with time spent surfing. Eventually, you'll be catching waves, dropping in, and hanging ten like the locals!

Bodyboarding is easier than surfing because you don't have to stand up. Instead, you surf a wave while lying on the board with your legs in the water. Before long, you can do huge wave-gouging turns or perform tricks such as an "El Rollo," a move where you roll into the lip of the wave and it rolls you over.

Waterskiing/Kneeboarding/Wakeboarding

The basic waterskiing principle is attitude: if you believe you can—you will! Remember learning to ride a bicycle? The hardest part was getting started. The bicycle was wobbly until you got going, and then it was easy to steer. It's the same with waterskiing. It's wobbly until you build up speed and get up on top of the water.

Waterskiing is a good water sport to learn if you want to kneeboard and wakeboard. You will learn much more easily if you already know how to water-ski.

To get started waterskiing, remember that safety is the most important thing—at all times. Everyone wants to be cool,

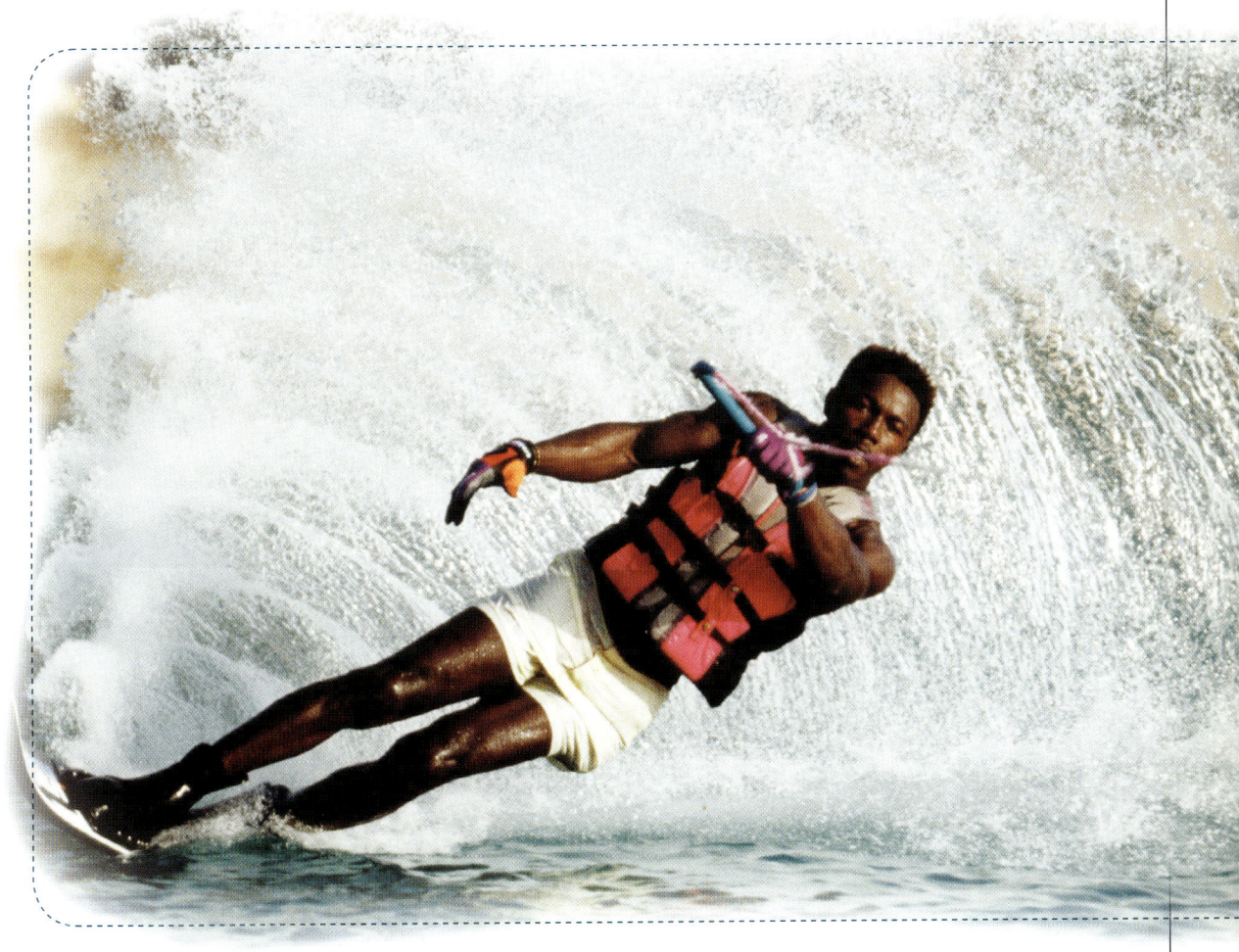

This water-skier kicks up a huge "roostertail" as he slices through the water at top speed.

but an accident or injury messes up everyone's good time. Make sure you always have a "spotter" in the boat—that's someone who is always watching the water-skier while the driver steers the boat.

The basic starting ski position is the cannonball—tucked with your hands around your legs. Stay that way in the water until the rope is tight and you're balanced. Then shout, "Hit It!" Stay tucked. The boat's speed will pull you out of the water; do not try to pull yourself up. In a few seconds, your skis will be on top of the water and you'll just need to stand up. Do so with straight arms, straight back, and bent knees. You'll probably fall down your first few tries. Don't worry about it. The boat will come around again and hook you up for another try.

Once you're up, use hand signals to communicate because the people on the boat won't be able to hear you. For instance:

- Thumbs up means faster.
- Thumbs down means slower.
- Patting your head means back to the dock.
- Holding up your arm when you fall means you're okay.
- A smile means you're having fun.

As the name implies, barefoot skiing is simply water-skiing without skis. Speed and calm water are the important factors. After you practice skiing barefoot, you can try some barefoot tricks, such as tumble turns, toe holds, toe turns, and 180- and 360-degree turns. Other types of skiing include **slalom,** trick, and jumping.

When kneeboarding, first place the board strap in the loosest position and make sure it is at the front of the kneepad. Lie on your stomach on the board. Signal the boat driver to take the speed up slowly. When the board begins to glide over the water, pull your knees onto the kneepad. Slowly slide or

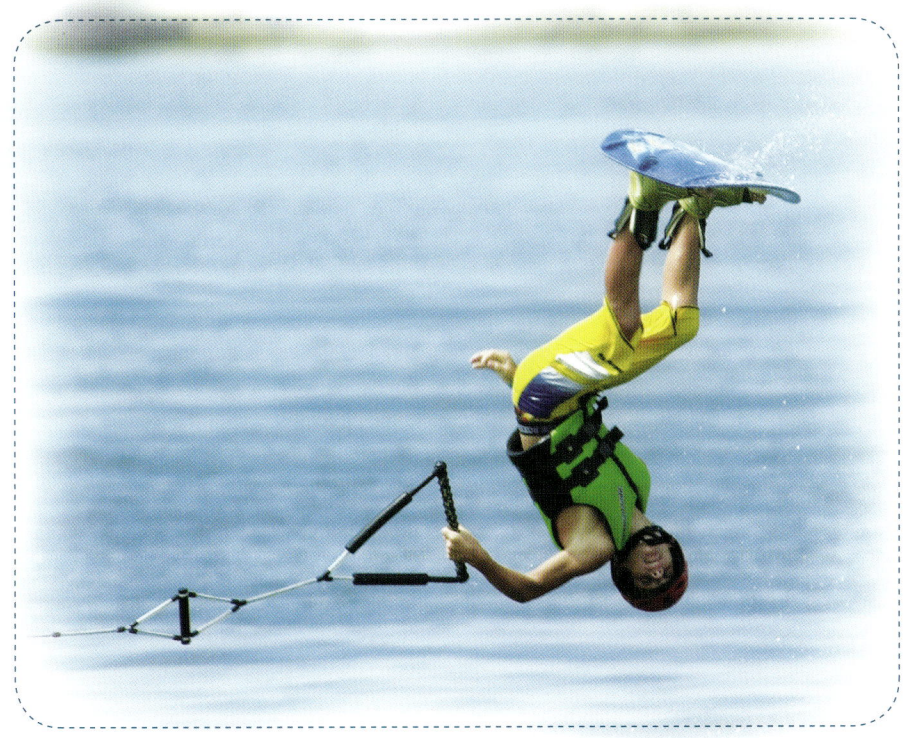

The special spinning wakeboard leash lets riders do amazing tricks such as this flip.

crawl on your knees until they reach the normal kneeling position. Once you are in a comfortable position, sit up, let go of the handle with one hand, and put the strap over your legs.

Wakeboarding is just as easy, but instead of kneeling on a board, you place your feet in straps and get pulled out of the water in the same fashion as you do when waterskiing. Riding a wakeboard, you will probably wonder what a half cab, indy, slob, roll to revert, tootsie roll, and slurpee all have in common? No, they're not treats you can buy at the 7-Eleven. This is wakeboard lingo for some of the most common tricks performed today. As you get better, you'll be doing some of them yourself.

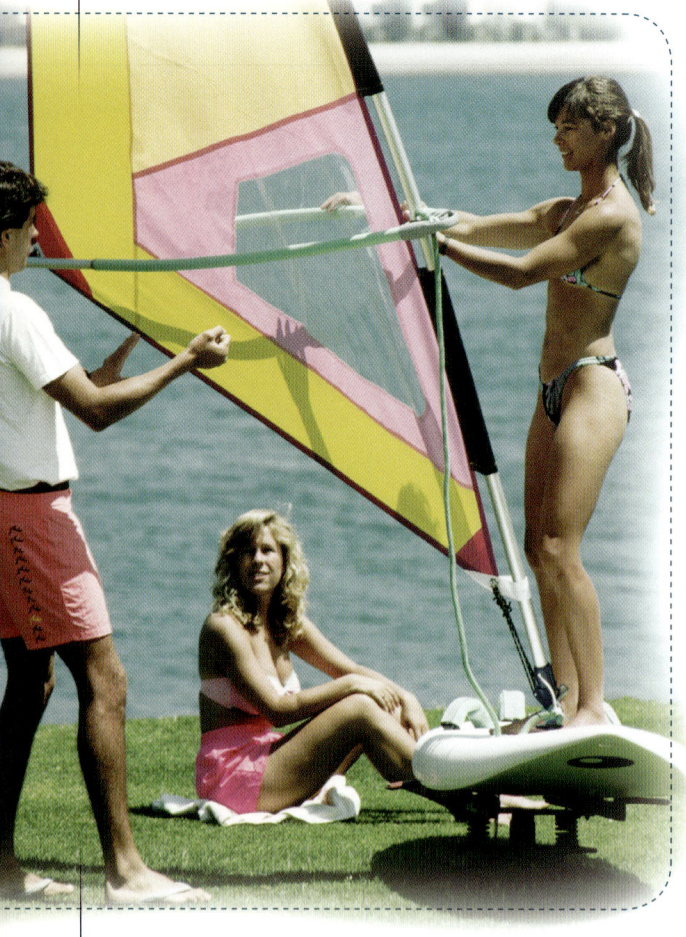

Practicing handling the windsurfer on land is the key to learning this fun but tricky sport.

Windsurfing/ Kitesurfing/ Hydrofoil Surfing

You should learn how to windsurf before attempting to kitesurf or hydrofoil surf. The best places to do all three of these have a combination of open beaches and windy weather.

To windsurf, always keep the **mast** upright. Practice holding the wishbone (the control bar attached to the mast) with one hand, while pulling in and releasing the sail with your other hand. Do this while the board is still on the beach or shore. This way you will get a good feel for the sail. After learning the sail movements onshore, practice "feeling" the balance of your board on the water.

Standing on the board, raise the sail and let it flap in the wind. Take the time to get your balance. Keeping the sail out of the water, lean the sail slightly back and forth, left to right, to learn how to position it. To start sailing, tilt the mast forward on your board and pull in the sail with your rear hand. To turn

HOW TO PERFORM A WINDSURFING BODY DRAG

Going full speed into the wind, take your front foot out of the footstrap and let it touch the water's surface. Your foot will immediately be pulled to the back. Then take your back foot out of the rear strap, lean to the back, and put that foot into the water. Bend your arms as much as possible. That gives you greater control over the sail. Your whole body should now be stretched so that only the lower part of your legs touch the water.

toward the wind, tilt the mast backward. To turn away from the wind, tilt the mast forward. Now you know the basics. With plenty of practice, you can join the pros in attempting such stunts as the air jibe, heli tack, body drag, 360, chop hop, and speed loop.

Kitesurfing is a cross between windsurfing and wakeboarding. Kitesurfers control a big wing made of lightweight fabric (the kite), which pulls them across or above the water. Most beginners travel downwind until they develop the skills for going upwind. Kitesurfers often do downwind runs, then hitch a ride back upwind to do it again.

In hydrofoil surfing—or foilboarding—the object is to glide above the water's surface so you hardly ever touch the water! Experiencing this "waterless" feeling is the sensation of a lifetime.

CHAPTER four

STARS AND COMPETITION

Imagine that, instead of being a teacher

or a lawyer, your job is to surf or water-ski. Sounds like a fun way to make money, doesn't it? But don't think it's easy. The world's best athletes have spent many years practicing. Most of them began when they were young boys and girls.

Let's take a look at some of the best men and women in water sports today.

Surfing/Bodyboarding

Six-time world champion Kelly Slater is perhaps the greatest surfer ever. This Floridian has won hundreds of thousands of dollars in prize money from surfing, and earns $1 million a year

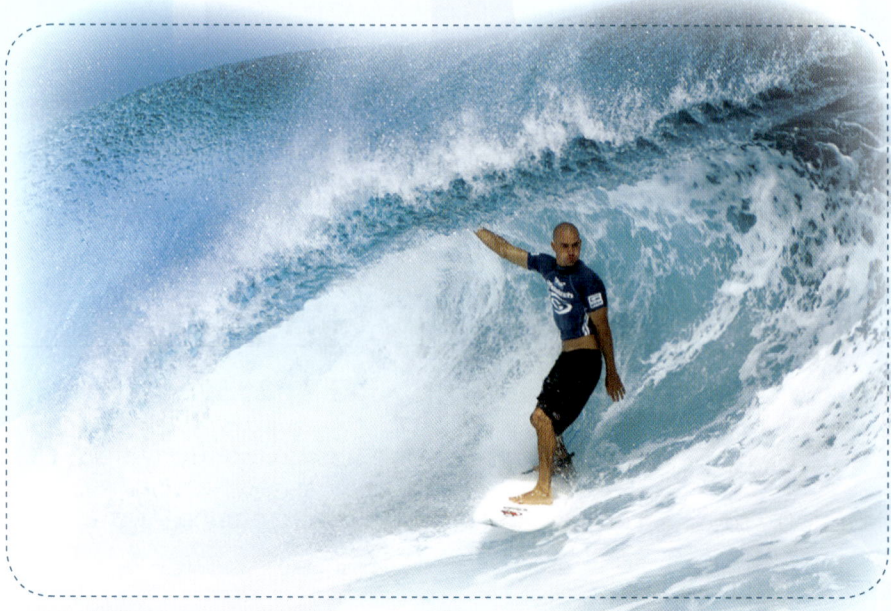

World champion surfer Kelly Slater shows how the pros "catch the curl," riding ahead of the breaking wave.

in **sponsorships!** He has surfed all over the world and has captured many top world titles.

Andy Irons from Hawaii is always ranked among the world's best surfers. Irons is one of the top surfers on the Association of Surfing Professionals (ASP) World Tour. In the world tour, surfers travel around the world to compete against each other. Irons was the 2002 and 2003 world champion. One of the best female wave-riders is six time world champion Layne Beachley. Fearless in big waves, Beachley has taken women's surfing to new heights in the last 10 years.

If you want to enter a surfing competition, there are amateur programs such as the National Scholastic Surfing Association and the Eastern Surfing Association. Young surfers from any state can compete and build skills to compete professionally.

If bodyboarding is your sport, the Atlantic Bodyboard Association is one place to look for upcoming competitions, tours, and the world's best. Some of the names to follow are Mike Stewart, Brian Myers, and Brian Mederios.

Waterskiing/Kneeboarding/Wakeboarding

Waterskiing is very popular, and USA Water Ski offers more than 800 tournaments a year. These range from local events for beginners to national and world-level tournaments for expe-

She's only 16, but Dallas Friday is among the world's best wakeboarders.

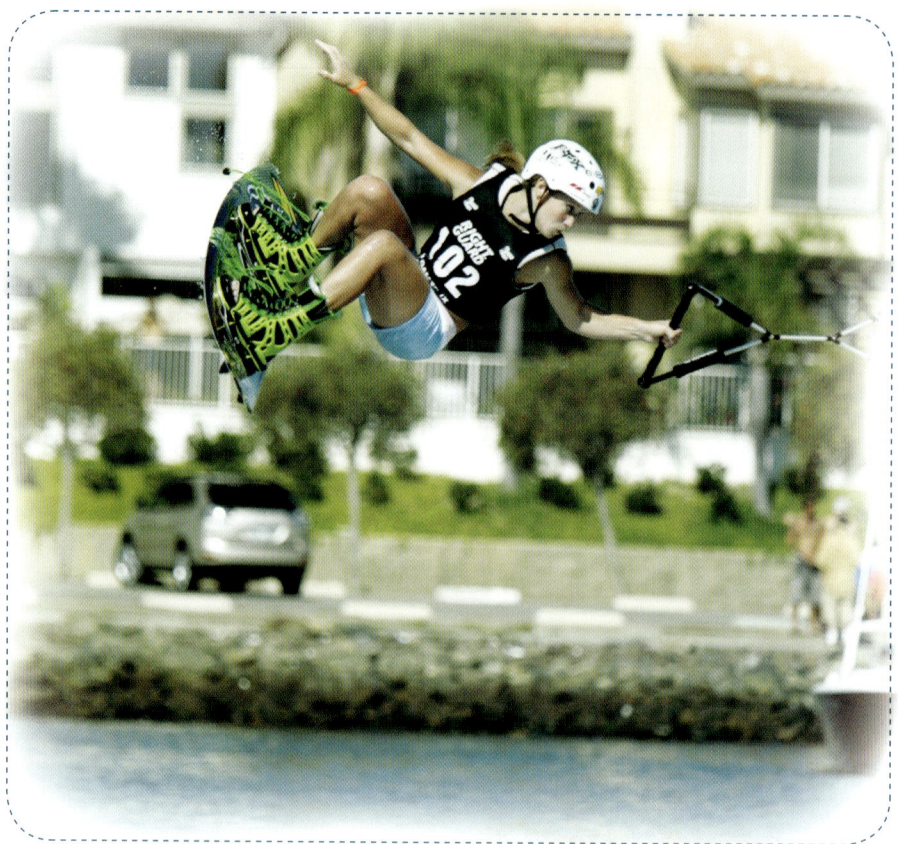

rienced competitors. Male and female skiers of all ages can compete in three events: slalom, tricks, and jumping. There are also events for barefoot, kneeboard, show-ski, ski-race, wakeboard, and physically challenged skiers.

Some of the world champions in waterskiing are Andy Mapple and Karen Truelove (slalom), Nicolas Le Forestier and Regina Jaquess (tricks), Jaret Llewellyn and Elena Milakova (jumping), and Keith St. Onge and Rachel George (barefoot). For kneeboarders, look out for Kenny Sanchez, Austin Hair, Natalie

Hair, and Trisha Rogerson. They are kids who are champions in the sport. Eric Voisin and Lisa Caldes are two of the biggest names among adult pros.

The ultimate titles for wakeboarding are the Pro Wakeboard Tour, the Vans Triple Crown of Wakeboarding, and the Wakeboard World Cup. J. D. Webb and Devin Rogers have been the two to beat in the boys division, while Darin Shapiro and Emily Copeland have won adult wakeboarding championships. Wakeboard star Dallas Friday is only 16, but already she has won many championships and even invented tricks!

Windsurfing/Kitesurfing/ Hydrofoil Surfing

Did you know that windsurfing is one of the few water sports where competitions can be held indoors? One such event in London, England, is held in a giant, indoor pool!

Windsurfing champs include Sam Ireland and Nikola Girke, while Dorota Staszewska of Poland is the women's World Cup champion. To prove that teenagers can compete with adults, 16-year-old Amy Carter of London came into the Canadian National Windsurf Championships as the World Youth Champion. This was her first competition against adult women, and she placed fifth.

For those wanting something different, kitesurfing offers exciting challenges on the professional level. In fact, many windsurfers also compete in world-class kitesurfing events. Eliot Leboe and Sierra Emory are professional windsurfers turned kitesurfers. Windsurfing legend Robby Naish has also been converted. Other big names in the sport include Cory Roeseler—

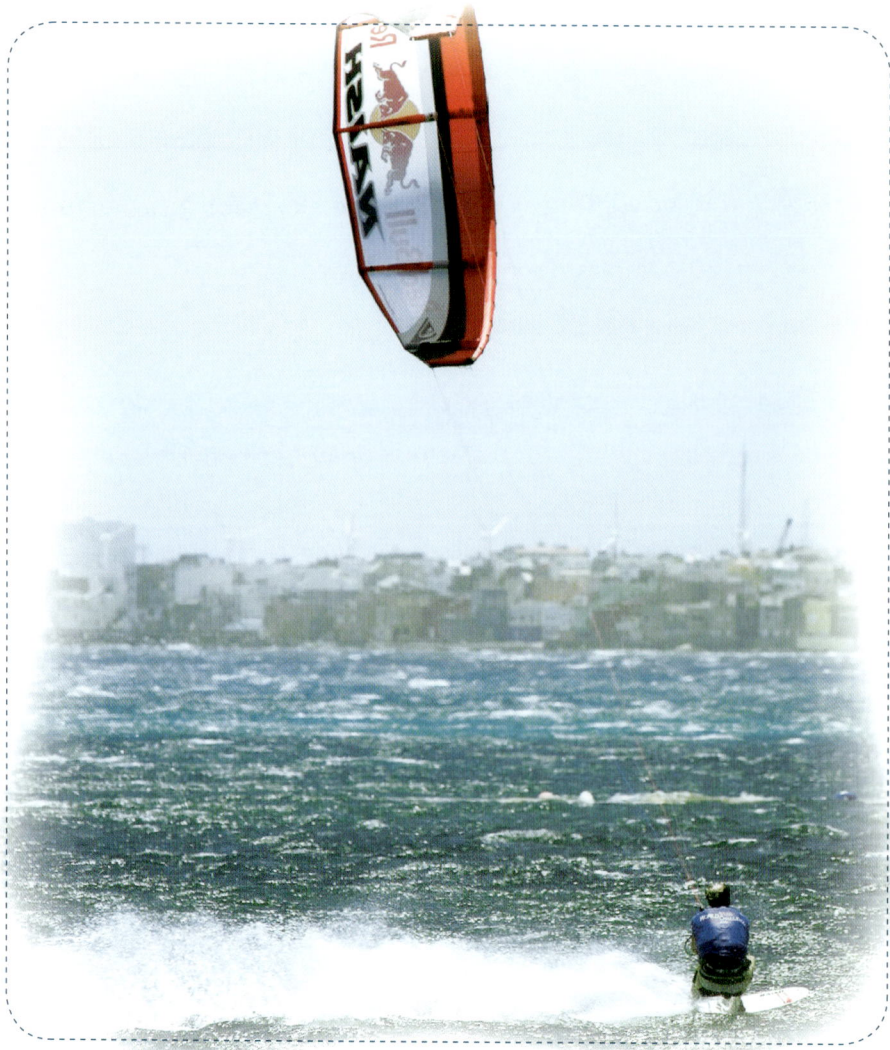

Former windsurfing champion Robbie Naish shows off his new passion: kitesurfing.

one of the inventors of kitesurfing—and sail designer Joe Koehl, who is responsible for getting kitesurfing up and running.

Hydrofoiling, like kitesurfing, is another popular water sport. World-class competitions such as the Air Chair Regatta showcase the best hydrofoil surfers and help this new sport grow. Some of the exciting pros are Geno Yauchler, Cameron Starks, and Ben Ferney.

No matter what type of water sport you choose, you're sure to find a way to compete if you want. Plus, you can look to the stars (on the water, that is, not in the sky!) for great examples to follow. Be safe, have fun, and get wet!

KITESURFERS MAKE HISTORY!

Kitesurfing is one of the newest extreme water sports. It takes great skill to guide the kite high above the waves as you zoom across the water's surface. The sport can take a lot out of you, so these surfers usually keep their rides short and sweet.

But three riders from Florida—Neal Hutchinson, Fabrice Collard, and Kent Marinkovic—apparently don't mind having sore arms. In December 2001, they set a record for nonstop kitesurfing.

Taking off from Key West, Florida (the southernmost point in the continental United States), they kitesurfed across the Florida Straits toward the island nation of Cuba. After 97 miles (156 km) and nine hours of nonstop kitesurfing, they made it! Despite rough seas, high winds, lack of food and water, and the chilling ocean, the surfers set a new kitesurfing distance world record!

GLOSSARY

buoyant —Having the ability to float in water.

catamaran —A boat with twin hulls connected by a deck.

drift —To be carried along by the wind or water.

hydrofoil —A boat with ski-like attachments at the front and back used to lift the front of the boat out of the water. The same concept was applied to the sit-down hydrofoil.

life vest —A jacket that can save a person from drowning by making them float.

mast —The vertical pole that supports a sail.

skin cancer —A dangerous skin condition that can kill you.

slalom —A zigzag course designed for ski racers.

sponsorships —Deals usually given to an athlete or celebrity in which they endorse a certain product in exchange for money.

stamina —The ability to not get tired.

wake —The path a boat leaves through the water, usually a pair of small waves moving in opposite directions.

water current —Water that moves all the time in a certain direction.

FIND OUT MORE

On the Web

Visit our home page for lots of links about water sports:
http://www.childsworld.com/links.html

NOTE TO PARENTS, TEACHERS, AND LIBRARIANS: We routinely check our Web links to make sure they're safe, active sites—so encourage your readers to check them out!

Books

Barker, Amanda. *Windsurfing.* Chicago: Heinemann Library, 2000.

Favret, Ben. *Complete Guide to Water Skiing.* Champaign, Ill.: Human Kinetics, 1997.

Werner, Doug. *Surfer's Start-Up: A Beginner's Guide to Surfing.* Ventura, Calif.: Pathfinder Publishing of California, 1993.

INDEX

Air Chair Regatta, 29
Association of Surfing Professionals (ASP), 25
Atlantic Bodyboard Association, 25

barefoot skiing, 6, 20
Beachley, Layne, 25
Bertin, Manu, 10
body drags, 23
bodyboarding, 11–12, 13, 18, 25

Canadian National Windsurfing Championships, 27
Carter, Amy, 27
competitions, 4, 25–26, 27, 29

Darby, Newman, 8
Drake, Jim, 8–9

"El Rollo," 18

Finn, Tony, 7
fins, 13
flysurfing, 9
foamies, 11
foilboarding. See hydrofoil surfing.
freeboarding, 6–7
Friday, Dallas, 27

Hamilton, Laird, 10
hand signals, 20
Hawaii, 10
hydrofoil surfing, 10, 15, 22, 23, 29

Irons, Andy, 25

Kahanamoku, Duke, 10
KiteSki system, 9
kitesurfing, 9–10, 14–15, 22, 23, 28–29
kneeboarding, 14, 18, 20–21, 26–27
Koehl, Joe, 29

leashes, 12
Legaignoux brothers, 9

lessons, 4, 11
life vests, 13, 15
lingo, 21

Mederios, Brian, 25
Murphy, Mike, 10
Myers, Brian, 25

National Scholastic Surfing Association, 25

partners, 16
Pope, Dick, Jr., 6
Pro Wakeboard Tour, 27

Roeseler, Cory, 9, 28–29

safety, 15, 18–19
Samuelson, Ralph, 6
Schweitzer, Hoyle, 9
ski rope, 13
skurfing. See wakeboarding.
Slater, Kelly, 24–25
speedboats, 13
Staszewska, Dorota, 27
Stewart, Mike, 25
surf wax, 12, 17
surfing, 10, 11–12, 16–18, 24–25

traction pads, 12
tricks, 6, 8, 13, 18, 20, 21, 23

USA Water Ski, 25

Vans Triple Crown of Wakeboarding, 27

Wakeboard World Cup, 27
wakeboarding, 7–8, 14, 18, 21, 27
Waller, Fred, 6
water currents, 16
waterskiing, 6, 13, 18–20, 25–26
wet suits, 12–13
windsurfing, 9, 14, 22–23, 27
Woolley, Bob, 10

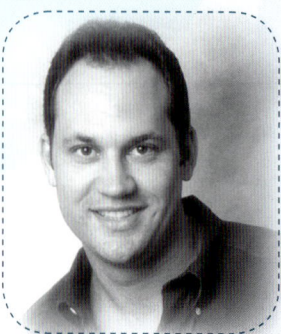

About the Author

James O. Fraioli grew up on Lake Washington in Bellevue, Washington, where he learned to water-ski, kneeboard, and wakeboard at an early age. His devotion to water sports continues to this day. Fraioli lives in Santa Barbara, California, and writes for *Santa Barbara Magazine*, *Seasons*, and *Dining & Destinations*.